W0106464

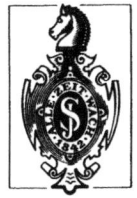

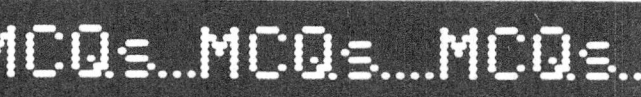
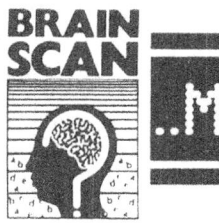

Roger Allen

Dermatology

Springer-Verlag
London Berlin Heidelberg New York
Paris Tokyo Hong Kong

Bernard Roger Allen, MB ChB, FRCP
Consultant Dermatologist, Department of Dermatology,
University Hospital, Queen's Medical Centre,
Nottingham NG7 2UH, UK

Publisher's note: The "Brainscan" logo is reproduced by courtesy of
The Editor, *Geriatric Medicine*, Modern Medicine GB Ltd.

ISBN-13:978-3-540-19607-5   e-ISBN-13:978-1-4471-1772-8
DOI: 10.1007/978-1-4471-1772-8

British Library Cataloguing in Publication Data
Allen, Roger, 1940–
Dermatology.
1. Medicine. Dermatology I. Title   616.5
ISBN-13:978-3-540-19607-5

Library of Congress Cataloging–in–Publication Data
Allen, Roger, 1940–
Dermatology/Roger Allen.
p. cm.
ISBN-13:978-3-540-19607-5
1. Dermatology—Examinations, questions, etc. I. Title.
[DNLM: 1. Skin Diseases—examination questions. WR 18 A428d]
RL74.2.A44 1990 616.5'0076—dc20 DNLM/DLC
for Library of Congress   90–9651
                                                                    CIP

Typeset by Photo·graphics, Honiton, Devon

2128/3916–543210 Printed on acid-free paper

Preface

Dermatology is a fascinating subject. This is a statement you might expect from a dermatologist, but what is the justification? It is a highly clinical specialty and sophisticated techniques of diagnosis are very much of secondary importance compared with clinical skills. The skin is important not only as an organ with vital physiological functions but also as a flag by which we communicate with the outside world. A perfect skin is desired by all, and upon this wish is based the multi-million pound cosmetics industry. Skin disease therefore places a strain on sufferers out of proportion to the disturbances in function which the pathology produces. A "leper" complex is frequent, and social and sexual contact may be shunned because of the embarrassment caused. It is also easy to overlook the contribution that cutaneous physical signs make towards diagnoses of internal disorders. Even straightforward factors such as the pallor of anaemia, the icterus of biliary obstruction or, quite simply, the age and sex of the patient are recognised immediately from visible signs in the skin. Like most other organs the skin has a limited repertoire of reactions, but these can occur in patients of all ages, combined together in an almost infinite number of permutations; hence the fascination referred to above.

It has been estimated that 10% of consultations with general practioners are because of a skin-related problem, and therefore a working knowledge of dermatology is essential for anyone who has regular clinical contact with patients. This book is aimed not only at medical students but also at those undertaking a VTS course for general practice or studying for the MRCP diploma, for whom it should provide a useful revision guide.

Nottingham   Roger Allen
1989

How to Use This Book

As a method of examination the use of multiple choice questions is likely to be a permanent and expanding feature on the educational scene. MCQs have their critics, but because of the wide range of topics which can be covered in one paper, and the ease with which responses can be marked by computer and analysed for effectiveness using such systems as the Kuder–Richardson reliability index, they have, in many fields, replaced more traditional examinations. They also lend themselves admirably to an efficient method of revision, and that is what has prompted this series of MCQs in dermatology.

There is no doubt that the best method of revision is not to read repeatedly through notes or texts but to answer questions ("What are the clinical features of Ehlers–Danlos syndrome?" "What are the symptoms of acute vitamin A toxicity?"). An attempt to apply a combination of knowledge and logic to a *question* followed then by reference to a book or notes will fix the subject in the mind to a degree surpassed only by having to carry out the same exercise in front of others. (To make a mistake in public greatly sharpens the mind.) It is with this approach that this series of multiple choice questions should be tackled. By considering and working through the 200 stems and 1000 suggested answers contained in this book it should be possible to acquire a reasonable basic grounding in the field of dermatology.

Many of the questions have been derived from a series of examination papers developed to assess the students at Nottingham University Medical School, where a two-month attachment to the Department of Dermatology is part of the middle-year curriculum. Most of the questions can be answered with a knowledge of one of the shorter undergraduate textbooks such as *Essentials of Dermatology* by J.L. Burton (Churchill Livingstone) or *Clinical Dermatology: Illustrated Textbook* by R.M. Mackie (Oxford University Press), but not all of them. There has to be an element of challenge, and reference to a larger work such as *Textbook of Dermatology* edited by A. Rook, D.S. Wilkinson, F.J.G. Ebling and J.L. Burton (Blackwell Scientific Publications) may occasionally be required.

Each question consists of a stem followed by five statements, none of which derives from or excludes any of the others. At least one correct and one incorrect answer follows each stem. A correct answer, either true or false, should be scored as +1, an abstention as 0 and an incorrect answer as −1.

Two medical aphorisms are that one should never say "Never" and that the more one knows about a subject the more difficult it is to give a straight "Yes" or "No" answer to a multiple choice question. Bear this in mind and use these questions sensibly, without looking for tricks and without believing that you should know about every exception to the general rule. It is worth remembering that examiners setting MCQs will tend to give false examples that are well outside the normal findings so that there can be less argument about whether the response is correct or not.

Go through the papers with a friend and argue about the answers – it is a good way to learn and can be fun, though that might depend on the friend. General guidelines for answering these and other MCQs are:

1. Read the question carefully. This seems obvious but it is often a source of simple mistakes. For example, is the question asking for a positive or a negative answer ("All 'x' do show 'y'" or "All 'x' do not show 'y'")? After reading the stem it is worth thinking about the topic for a moment or two before looking at the alternatives presented. For example, if the stem says "In basal cell carcinomata . . ." think briefly about what you know about the lesions. Then look at what is given; some of the things you have thought about may be in front of you.

2. Do not guess. Most multiple choice wrong answers are included because they have a certain familiar ring about them;

they are close to the truth but not quite close enough. Therefore, if you are totally ignorant about a subject do not try to answer the questions.

3. Be decisive. If you think an answer is correct mark it as such and move on. If you spend too long on thinking about an answer you can almost always persuade yourself that it is right, or wrong as the case may be.

4. If the answer is not obvious after careful reading miss the question out and come back to it at the end.

5. Ignore statistics. Just answer each question as it is set and do not try to work on the basis either of how many marks you have already scored or how many right or wrong answers have been presented.

The questions in this book have been divided into 10 revision papers of 20 questions each. Each paper covers a wide range of topics. Many of the answers are followed by brief explanatory comments, but when tackling the questions it is a good idea to have a textbook to hand so that you can carry out further reading on an immediate basis whilst the subject is still fresh in your mind.

Contents

Paper 1

Q.1.1   Psoriasis

a. may involve the external auditory meatus
b. is likely to be more severe if close relatives have the disease
c. may be associated with an ankylosing spondylitis type of arthritis
d. can cause actual disappearance of the phalanges
e. occurs in a pustular form only on the hands and feet

Q.1.2   Neurofibromatosis

a. is an autosomal recessive condition
b. may start with café au lait patches
c. produces characteristic hard nodules in the skin
d. usually first becomes evident at the time of puberty
e. is a cosmetic problem only in the vast majority of patients

Q.1.3   Purpura may be a feature of

a. Henoch–Schönlein disease
b. excessive use of 1% hydrocortisone
c. lichen planus
d. amyloidosis
e. a positive Hess test

Q.1.4   Venous insufficiency of the lower limb

a. is always the result of damage to the veins
b. causes an eczema in most cases
c. is defined as occurring when tissue osmotic pressure exceeds venous capillary pressure
d. may produce "atrophie blanche" even in the absence of ulceration
e. may damage the muscles

For answers see over

Answers

A.1.1 a. T—It is one cause of otitis externa.
      b. F—The likelihood of developing the disorder is increased but the severity is independent of this factor.
      c. T
      d. T—"Acro-osteolysis" is the most severe form of the disease.
      e. T—Pustulation can be widespread.

A.1.2 a. F—It is autosomal dominant.
      b. T—More than six patches in an infant is suggestive.
      c. F—The nodules are very typically soft.
      d. F—In 80% of cases there is some evidence before puberty.
      e. T—Complications occur in only 10% of cases.

A.1.3 a. T—Nodular purpura around the ankles is a typical feature.
      b. F—This preparation is too weak to cause the purpura seen with stronger fluorinated preparations.
      c. F
      d. T—Amyloid deposits cause weakness in the vascular wall.
      e. T—By definition.

A.1.4 a. F—Simple immobility, e.g. from osteoarthritis, will also cause venous insufficiency of the lower limb.
      b. F—Most of the eczema is due to therapy.
      c. F—Venous insufficiency of the lower limb occurs when venous pressure exceeds tissue osmotic pressure.
      d. T
      e. T—The same destructive process is going on in the other tissues of the limb.

Questions

Q.1.5 Acne

a. affects the face more commonly than any other area
b. never spreads as far as the buttocks
c. in a 12-month-old infant is likely to indicate an endocrine upset
d. tends to resolve at an earlier age in females than males
e. may be caused by systemic prednisolone therapy

Q.1.6 UVB is suitable treatment for

a. vitiligo
b. pityriasis versicolor
c. acne vulgaris
d. psoriasis
e. atopic eczema

Q.1.7 Chronic ulceration of the lower limb may occur in

a. Felty's syndrome
b. arterial insufficiency
c. diabetes
d. ichthyosis
e. chronic lymphoedema

Q.1.8 In disorders of lipid metabolism

a. eruptive xanthomata may be a sign of diabetes
b. xanthelasmata respond to lowering the blood cholesterol
c. hypothyroidism is associated with a lowered blood cholesterol
d. tendon xanthomata are typical of secondary causes
e. eruptive xanthomata are rapidly reversible

Q.1.9 Pruritus is a not infrequent feature of

a. pityriasis rosea
b. pityriasis versicolor
c. secondary syphilis
d. alopecia areata
e. polycythaemia rubra vera

For answers see over

Answers

A.1.5 a. T
      b. F—In severe cases it may spread as far as the thighs.
      c. F—At this age infantile acne may be evident.
      d. T—The median ages for maximum frequency are 17 years in females and 19 years in males.
      e. F—Unlike idiopathic Cushing's disease.

A.1.6 a. F—There is no evidence that UVB helps, but PUVA has been used.
      b. F
      c. T—It can have a marked effect on the inflammatory component.
      d. T
      e. F—But here again PUVA has been claimed to be beneficial.

A.1.7 a. T—Rheumatoid arthritis with hypersplenism and neutropenia.
      b. T—Often with severe pain.
      c. T—Usually trophic and therefore on the foot.
      d. F
      e. T—Multiple small chronically weeping ulcers are frequently seen.

A.1.8 a. T—They are a feature of uncontrolled diabetes mellitus.
      b. F—They rarely improve.
      c. F—The cholesterol is typically raised.
      d. F—They are found in primary metabolic disorders of lipid metabolism.
      e. T—They disappear quickly when the cause is corrected.

A.1.9 a. T—But it occurs in well under half of sufferers.
      b. F—Only exceptionally rarely.
      c. F
      d. F
      e. T

Q.1.10 It is true to state that

  a. albinism is due to a congenital lack of melanocytes
  b acne may be particularly severe in epileptics
  c. blue naevi are premalignant
  d. chilblains in children are often followed by Raynaud's phenomenon in adult life
  e. cranial arteritis may give ulceration of the scalp

Q.1.11 The individual lesions of urticaria

  a. are due mainly to the local release of histamine
  b. fade within 24 hours of their appearance
  c. may leave slight residual scaling
  d. are always triggered by slight trauma (dermatographia)
  e. vary considerably in area

Q.1.12 Nails

  a. may thicken as a result of trauma
  b. may become white in renal failure
  c. show splinter haemorrhages in psoriasis
  d. show longitudinal ridging following a debilitating illness
  e. are softer than normal in psoriasis

Q.1.13 Allergic contact dermatitis

  a. is due to type 1 hypersensitivity
  b. is often induced by rubber latex
  c. due to nickel is more common in women than men
  d. shows increased frequency in patients with gravitational leg ulcers
  e. may be treated with topical tar preparations

Q.1.14 Seborrhoeic dermatitis in infants

  a. may cause cradle cap
  b. is a synonym for napkin dermatitis
  c. is due to ammonia formed by the breakdown of urine on a nappy
  d. may develop later into atopic dermatitis
  e. responds to topical antibiotics

For answers see over

Answers

A.1.10 a. F—There is a lack of tyrosinase, but the number of melanocytes is normal.
b. T—Possibly due to anticonvulsant therapy.
c. F—They are benign pigmented naevi of the deep dermis.
d. F
e. T

A.1.11 a. T
b. T—Often within a couple of hours.
c. F—The skin surface is always normal.
d. F—This is just one cause.
e. T—Possibly linked to depth, with more extensive lesions being deeper.

A.1.12 a. T—If the nail matrix is damaged.
b. F—Leukonychia is a feature of liver failure with hypoalbuminaemia.
c. T—These are distally situated and of traumatic origin.
d. F—The ridges are transverse (Beau's lines).
e. F—But soft keratin may accumulate subungually.

A.1.13 a. F—Type 4 cell-mediated hypersensitivity.
b. F—Pure latex rarely sensitizes, it is the other ingredients of rubber than cause problems.
c. T—Due to greater exposure, e.g. brassière clips and cheap jewellery.
d. T—Due to greater exposure to medicaments and predisposition of the limb because of venous insufficiency.
e. F—Tar preparations tend to irritate exogenous eczema.

A.1.14 a. T—A common presenting feature.
b. F—It is just one cause of a napkin eruption.
c. F—Decomposing urine on a nappy is the cause of ammoniacal napkin dermatitis.
d. F—The two conditions are separate.
e. F—Combinations of mild steroids and antiseptics with an activity against candida are most effective.

Q.1.15 Recognised cutaneous signs of internal malignancy include

a. acanthosis nigricans
b. dermatomyositis
c. lichen planus
d. acquired ichthyosis
e. Campbell de Morgan spots

Q.1.16 Invasive squamous cell carcinoma of the skin

a. is commonest on the trunk
b. can arise at sites of previous lupus vulgaris
c. may be an industrial disease
d. should be treated by excision
e. usually metastasises early

Q.1.17 Cutaneous leishmaniasis

a. is a mild form of visceral leishmaniasis
b. causes a chronic non-healing ulcer which lasts about a year
c. may be acquired on a Mediterranean holiday
d. results in slow systemic spread
e. is spread by ticks

Q.1.18 Of infestations it is true to say that

a. bedbugs live in the seams of clothing
b. malathion is a suitable treatment for head lice
c. in body lice infestations the clothes should be incinerated
d. pubic lice only affect adults
e. cat flea bites are usually restricted to the legs

Q.1.19 Diphtheroids contribute to the disease process in

a. chronic paronychia
b. pitted keratolysis
c. trichomycosis axillaris
d. acne vulgaris
e. rosacea

For answers see over

Answers

A.1.15 a. T—A benign form also exists, seen in the obese.
 b. T—In adults, but not in children.
 c. F
 d. T
 e. F

A.1.16 a. F—In the majority of cases it occurs on light-exposed areas of the body.
 b. T
 c. T—Historically, the incidence was high among chimney sweeps, but tar extracts are also carcinogenic.
 d. T
 e. F—Fortunately not.

A.1.17 a. F—The two are separate diseases.
 b. T
 c. T—It is patchily endemic on the Mediterranean littoral.
 d. F—It remains confined to the skin.
 e. F—It is spread by sand flies (commonly *Phlebotomus papatasii*).

A.1.18 a. F—They prefer to live between hard flat surfaces, e.g. behind pictures on the wall or in cracks in the bed frame.
 b. T—Also kills the unhatched eggs (nits).
 c. F—Thorough laundering is all that is required.
 d. F—They will affect the eyelashes of prepubertal children.
 e. T—Cats aren't very big and their fleas don't jump very high.

A.1.19 a. F—Candida is responsible.
 b. T—A diphtheroid infection of sweaty feet.
 c. T—Colonisation of axillary hairs.
 d. T—*Propionibacterium acnes* breaks down neutral lipids.
 e. F

Q.1.20 Scabies

a. is called sarcoptic mange when it occurs in animals
b is caused by a small insect which burrows into the epidermis
c. can be contracted from bedding
d. is treated by the daily application of benzyl benzoate emulsion until the itching ceases
e. may become secondarily infected

For answers see over

Answers

A.1.20 a. T

      b. F—*Sarcoptes scabiei* var. *hominis* is a small mite – an eight-legged arthropod.

      c. F—Skin-to-skin contact is necessary.

      d. F—The preparation is effective after a single application. It is highly irritating and continuation of treatment will cause dermatitis.

      e. T

Paper 2

Q.2.1 Regarding the case of a 70-year-old man who developed a tumour on his cheek with a central keratin plug. It had grown rapidly for 8 weeks to 3.0 cm in diameter before showing signs of regression:

    a. This history is suggestive of a basal cell carcinoma
    b. Early excision is to be advised to prevent metastases
    c. Treatment with curettage will be adequate
    d. Biopsy of the edge will clearly differentiate it from a squamous cell carcinoma
    e. Spontaneous resolution will occur if it is left alone

Q.2.2 Seborrhoeic dermatitis

    a. causes dandruff when the scalp is affected
    b. may affect the eyelashes
    c. has a similar histology to psoriasis
    d. responds readily to mild topical steroids
    e. can be treated with systemic tetracycline

Q.2.3 Scabies is

    a. most common in Norway
    b. due just to the female mite
    c. usually the result of infestation with fewer than 12 mites
    d. now resistant to gammabenzene hexachloride
    e. commoner in patients with Down's syndrome

Q.2.4 Mycobacteria are responsible for

    a. lupus vulgaris
    b. fish tank granuloma
    c. acrodermatitis continua
    d. erythrasma
    e. buruli ulcer

Q.2.5 An autosomal dominant inheritance occurs in

    a. psoriasis
    b. tuberous sclerosis
    c. ichthyosis vulgaris
    d. atopic eczema
    e. all forms of epidermolysis bullosa

For answers see over

Answers

A.2.1 a. F—It is typical of a keratoacanthoma.
     b. F—It does not metastasise.
     c. T
     d. F—Biopsy of the edge of the tumour is not a reliable method of differential diagnosis.
     e. T—But with scarring.

A.2.2 a. T—Dandruff is the commonest presenting feature.
     b. T—Blepharitis is frequent, particularly in children.
     c. F
     d. F—The response is often poor and temporary.
     e. F

A.2.3 a. F—The term "Norwegian scabies" refers to a severe non-itchy form that occurs in immunosuppressed patients.
     b. T—Only the female burrows; the males live on the skin surface around hair follicles.
     c. T—Not all visible lesions contain mites.
     d. F—This remains an effective and relatively non-irritating treatment.
     e. T—And other mentally defective patients.

A.2.4 a. T—This is tuberculosis of the skin.
     b. T—This and swimming pool granuloma are due to *M. balnei*.
     c. F—This is a chronic form of psoriasis.
     d. F—This is due to *Corynebacterium minutissimum*.
     e. T—This is due to *M. ulcerans*.

A.2.5 a. F—The exact mode of inheritance of the diathesis is unknown.
     b. T
     c. T
     d. F—The exact mode of inheritance is unknown.
     e. F—The most severe forms have a recessive inheritance.

Q.2.6 **Mast cells**

a. are more numerous in the lesions of urticaria
b. possess receptors for activation by IgE
c. contain heparin
d. release histamine more easily after aspirin treatment
e. are stabilised by the food dye tartrazine

Q.2.7 **Wood's light is useful in the diagnosis of**

a. tinea corporis
b. erythrasma
c. *Trichophyton rubrum* infections
d. some types of porphyria
e. epiloia

Q.2.8 **The following systemic antimicrobial therapies may be beneficial in acne:**

a. Erythromycin
b. Metronidazole
c. Co-trimoxazole
d. Amoxycillin
e. Doxycycline

Q.2.9 **Deficiency of**

a. zinc causes acrodermatitis enteropathica
b. vitamin C causes bone pain
c. protein causes kwashiorkor
d. vitamin A causes mouth ulcers
e. iron causes brittle nails

Q.2.10 **Adverse reations to drugs**

a. give an eczematous eruption most commonly
b. are said to be "fixed" if they occur each time the drug is given
c. are always based on an allergy
d. may resemble lichen planus
e. tend to increase in severity each time the drug is given

For answers see over

Answers

A.2.6 a. F
      b. T
      c. T
      d. T
      e. F—Tartrazine has a similar effect to aspirin.

A.2.7 a. F—Only helpful in tinea capitis where the terminal hairs may fluoresce.
      b. T—There is a coral pink fluorescence of the skin surface in this condition.
      c. F—This organism does not fluoresce even when affecting the scalp.
      d. T—For example, the extracted urine may fluoresce pink in acquired porphyria.
      e. T—The depigmented areas are more easily seen.

A.2.8 a. T
      b. F
      c. T
      d. F
      e. T

A.2.9 a. T—This is a classic deficiency disease caused by a defect in absorption of zinc.
      b. T—Bone pain is a prominent feature of scurvy.
      c. T—This is protein energy malnutrition.
      d. F
      e. T—In addition to koilonychia.

A.2.10 a. F—An eczema is rare.
      b. F—A fixed drug eruption occurs at the same site each time the drug is given.
      c. F—Many other mechanisms may be involved.
      d. T
      e. F—The same pattern is repeated each time.

Q.2.11 Common causes of erythema multiforme include

a. primary tuberculosis
b. streptococcal infections
c. orf
d. drugs
e. herpes zoster

Q.2.12 In urticaria

a. the irritation caused is made evident by widespread excoriations
b. the symptoms are best relieved by topical antihistamines
c. allergies are the commonest cause
d. spontaneous resolution occurs in most cases
e. patch tests are useful in elucidating a cause

Q.2.13 Alopecia areata

a. is the commonest cause of patchy scarring alopecia
b. affects only the scalp
c. is characterised by the presence of question mark hairs
d. retains the potential for regrowth in all cases
e. responds to systemic steroid therapy

Q.2.14 Insects are vectors for

a. bubonic plague
b. Lyme disease
c. cholera
d. leishmaniasis
e. AIDS

Q.2.15 Systemic diseases giving rise to generalised pruritus include

a. obstructive jaundice
b. systemic lymphoma
c. primary biliary cirrhosis
d. carcinoid syndrome
e. chronic adrenal failure

For answers see over

Answers

A.2.11 a. F—Erythema *nodosum* may occur.
      b. F—Erythema *nodosum* may occur.
      c. T—The commonest cause on an "at risk" basis.
      d. T
      e. F—Very unusual, unlike herpes simplex.

A.2.12 a. F—Excoriations are never present.
      b. T—Systemic antihistamines are the treatment of choice.
      c. F—Approximately 90% of cases are "idiopathic".
      d. T
      e. F—Scratch tests might identify an allergic cause, e.g. a food, but are rarely indicated in practice.

A.2.13 a. F—Patchy alopecia, yes, but scarring is not a feature.
      b. F—Any hair-bearing area of the body may be involved.
      c. F—Exclamation mark hairs are characteristic.
      d. T—Even after many years of inactivity.
      e. T—But relapse occurs when it is withdrawn.

A.2.14 a. T—Rat fleas.
      b. T—Ticks.
      c. F
      d. T—Sand flies or mosquitoes.
      e. F—There is no evidence for spread by blood-sucking insects.

A.2.15 a. T
      b. T
      c. T—Often generalised pruritus is the earliest symptom.
      d. F
      e. F

Q.2.16 Atopic eczema

a. does not occur without associated asthma
b. can be excluded as a cause of eczema if the onset is in adult life
c. might be associated with reduced sensitivity to β-agonist stimuli
d. starts within 3 months of birth in most cases
e. should not be treated with topical steroids stronger than 1% hydrocortisone when it occurs in children

Q.2.17 Appropriate therapies include

a. dithranol preparations for chronic lichenified eczema
b. systemic steroids for dermatitis herpetiformis
c. antimalarials for discoid lupus erythematosus (DLE)
d. metronidazole for rosacea
e. tar for DLE

Q.2.18 Candida intertrigo can be distinguished from flexural psoriasis by

a. better symmetry
b. a less sharp margin to the lesion
c. the presence of candida on culture
d. the presence of satellite lesions
e. the degree of scaling

Q.2.19 Benign haemangiomata are

a. found in about 10% of middle-aged adults
b. a feature of AIDS
c. part of the Peutz–Jegher syndrome
d. frequent on the scrotum in elderly men
e. the source of haemorrhage in Osler–Rendu–Weber disease

Q.2.20 Infections contracted from animal sources include

a. orf
b. *Erysipelothrix rhusiopathiae* infection
c. *Microsporum audouinii* infection
d. scabies
e. *Trichophyton verrucosum* infection

For answers see over

Answers

A.2.16 a. F—Although the association is common.
  b. F—Although it is unusual.
  c. T
  d. F—The onset is usually after the age of 3 months and before the age of 2 years.
  e. F—Treatment should be prescribed according to disease severity not age, but the surface area to weight ratio is higher in children, and so systemic absorption of steroids is proportionately greater.

A.2.17 a. F—Dithranol is only useful for psoriasis.
  b. F—Dapsone is highly specific for this condition.
  c. T—Particularly effective for light sensitivity.
  d. T—The next choice if tetracycline fails.
  e. F

A.2.18 a. T—It affects moist areas which are likely to be symmetrical, e.g. under both breasts or both sides of the groin.
  b. T—Psoriasis retains its clear-cut margin.
  c. F—Candida is a frequent contaminant in flexural psoriasis.
  d. T
  e. F—Neither condition scales significantly.

A.2.19 a. F—Campbell de Morgan spots are almost universal.
  b. F—Malignant angiosarcomata occur.
  c. F—The perioral lesions are melanotic.
  d. T
  e. T—Synonym is hereditary *haemorrhagic* telangiectasia.

A.2.20 a. T—This is pustular contagious dermatitis of sheep (and goats).
  b. T—Particularly from pork.
  c. F—This fungus causes human scalp ringworm.
  d. F—Although contact with the animal equivalent, sarcoptic mange, may give local irritation.
  e. T—This organism is responsible for cattle ringworm.

Paper 3

Q.3.1 Lupus vulgaris

a. may be slowly progressive over 20 years or more
b. is due to primary tuberculosis of the skin
c. may be premalignant
d. produces violaceous plaques with "apple jelly" nodules on diascopy
e. is becoming more frequent again because of AIDS

Q.3.2 Increased pigmentation may result from

a. chronic renal failure
b. inflammation of the skin
c. hyperadrenalism
d. lichen planus
e. oral contraceptive therapy

Q.3.3 Cellulitis of the leg

a. starts in most cases with general malaise and rigors
b. can be treated with bed rest and elevation of the leg alone
c. is painful
d. may spread rapidly
e. does not ulcerate

Q.3.4 Benign cellular naevi (moles)

a. show some degree of pigmentation in all cases
b. are the commonest site for malignant melanoma to arise
c. are unusual before the age of 2 years
d. are more likely to become malignant if traumatised
e. are benign if they show a growth of terminal hairs

Q.3.5 Ichthyosis

a. occurs in a sex-linked form
b. gets its name from the slight fishy odour it produces
c. may be associated with atopic eczema
d. occurs occasionally as an acquired condition
e. should be treated by the application of very mild topical steroids

For answers see over

Answers

A.3.1 a. T
        b. F—It is post primary, hence the slow spread.
        c. T—Squamous cell carcinoma is a significant risk.
        d. T
        e. T—Although reactivation of old pulmonary tuberculosis does occur.

A.3.2 a. T
        b. T—So-called post inflammatory pigmentation.
        c. F—It is caused by *hypo*adrenalism (Addison's disease).
        d. T—Very common as resolution occurs.
        e. T—Chloasma is associated with oral contraceptives.

A.3.3 a. T—Before the symptoms and signs localise.
        b. F—Antibiotics are mandatory.
        c. T
        d. T—Treatment should therefore by initiated without delay.
        e. F—Ulceration may be severe and extensive if treatment has been inadequate.

A.3.4 a. F
        b. F—But melanomata may arise from dysplastic naevi and those showing junctional activity.
        c. T
        d. F—This is a rumour attributable to old wives.
        e. T

A.3.5 a. T—But the commonest form is autosomal dominant.
        b. F—The name comes from the characteristic scaliness.
        c. T
        d. T—Acquired ichthyosis is very rare and linked to malignancy.
        e. F—Steroids should not be used.

Q.3.6 Excessive sweating

a. may be an early symptom of phaeochromocytoma
b. is restricted to the axillae, palms and soles in thyrotoxicosis
c. when localised may be controlled by the application of aluminium chloride hexahydrate
d. of the palms can be relieved by cervical sympathectomy
e. can be controlled by the use of oral anticholinergic drugs

Q.3.7 Spider naevi

a. are physiological in children
b. increase in number in pregnancy
c. are confined to the upper half of the body
d. may be a sign of internal malignancy
e. increase in number in renal failure

Q.3.8 It is true to say that in patients with acne

a. greasy foods should be avoided
b. all blocked sebaceous glands show a blackhead
c. surgery is the treatment of choice for cysts
d. the cause is occasionally occupational
e. sexual malpractices may contribute to the problem

Q.3.9 Retinoids

a. are derivatives of vitamin D
b. are teratogenic
c. have largely replaced antibiotics as the systemic treatment of choice in acne
d. cause dryness of the lips as their most frequent side effect
e. are useful in the treatment of atopic eczema

Q.3.10 Generalised lymphadenopathy may be a feature of

a. impetigo
b. extensive atopic eczema
c. roseola infantum (exanthema subitum)
d. early HIV infection
e. erythema multiforme

For answers see over

Answers

A.3.6
a. T
b. F—With any metabolic cause it tends to be generalised.
c. T—This chemical is a common ingredient of antiperspirants.
d. T—But not recommended except in the most severe cases.
e. F—Although theoretically possible, intolerable side effects occur before control of the sweating is achieved.

A.3.7
a. T—Rare indeed is the child without at least one.
b. T—And resolve 6 weeks afterwards.
c. T—The drainage area of the superior vena cava.
d. F
e. F—But they do in liver failure.

A.3.8
a. F—There is no evidence that they are harmful.
b F—If the blockage is beneath the duct a closed comedo (whitehead) is formed.
c. F—Scarring will result.
d. T—Acne can be caused by mineral oil, tar or halogenated hydrocarbons.
e. F—An enduring myth which adds insult to an already injured psyche.

A.3.9
a. F—They are derivatives of vitamin A.
b. T—In the case of etretinate the teratogenic effect continues for up to 2 years after the last dose.
c. F
d. T
e. F

A.3.10
a. F—The infection is too superficial.
b. T—Even in the absence of overt infection.
c. F
d. T
e. F

Q.3.11 Rheumatoid nodules

    a. are confined to the hands and elbows
    b. may be found in severe psoriatic arthropathy
    c. may be the first manifestation of rheumatoid disease
    d. may ulcerate
    e. resolve on systemic steroid therapy

Q.3.12 Tattoos

    a. are readily removed by dermabrasion
    b. may indicate a risk of hepatitis
    c. may give rise to an allergic granuloma
    d. can be destroyed by CO_2 laser
    e. are the result of deposition of pigment in the epidermis

Q.3.13 The lesions of molluscum contagiosum

    a. are umbilicated papules
    b. may induce eczema in the surrounding skin
    c. are more frequent on exposed areas
    d. resolve following an inflammatory stimulus
    e. are unusual before the age of 5 years

Q.3.14 Erythema nodosum may be caused by

    a. sarcoidosis
    b. post primary tuberculosis
    c. ulcerative colitis
    d. staphylococcal infections
    e. herpes simplex

Q.3.15 Well-recognised causes of urticaria include:

    a. tartrazine allergy
    b. penicillin allergy
    c. contact dermatitis
    d. aspirin sensitivity
    e. exposure to cold

For answers see over

Answers

A.3.11 a. F—They may be very extensive.
  b. F—They are only found in latex-positive rheumatoid arthritis.
  c. T—Sometimes months before arthritis develops.
  d. T—This may indicate increased disease activity.
  e. F—Although they may improve slightly.

A.3.12 a. F—Tattoos are usually very difficult to remove; total excision may be required.
  b. T—Unsterile needles can transmit hepatitis.
  c. T—Due to the pigments used, particularly those containing mercury.
  d. T—Laser reatment is a reasonable alternative to surgery.
  e. F—The pigment is deposited in the dermis.

A.3.13 a. T
  b. T—This is quite common, especially in children.
  c. F—They are more common on covered areas.
  d. T—This is the rationale behind many forms of treatment, e.g. touching with phenol or cryotherapy.
  e. F—They are more common in young children.

A.3.14 a. T—Perhaps the most commonly identified cause.
  b. F—It occurs only in the primary phase.
  c. T—As well as other enteropathies.
  d. F—*Strepto*coccal infections are responsible.
  e. F—Erythema *multiforme* is the usual response.

A.3.15 a. F—Tartrazine acts as a histamine release agent not an allergen.
  b. T
  c. F—This is often an important differential diagnosis.
  d. T
  e. T—One of the physical causes.

Q.3.16 Hair growth

a. occurs from the hair papilla
b. changes from vellus to terminal under the influence of androgens
c. is nearly always without pigment in patches of vitiligo
d. around the breasts of females is a reliable sign of an endocrine abnormality
e. is most active during the catagen phase

Q.3.17 Contact dermatitis may be induced by handling

a. cobalt
b. chromate
c. mercury
d. silver
e. aluminium

Q.3.18 It is true to say of psoriasis that

a. topical steroids are the treatment of choice
b. it is unusual under the age of 10 years
c. it may cause a rheumatoid-factor positive arthropathy
d. a relapse may follow a streptococcal sore throat
e. it is associated with an increased familial incidence of asthma and hay fever

Q.3.19 A keratoacanthoma

a. may be indistinguishable histologically from a squamous cell carcinoma
b. may be clinically indistinguishable from a basal cell carcinoma (BCC)
c. grows for a year then slowly resolves
d. usually shows telangiectasia
e. is a highly malignant tumour

Q.3.20 Erythrasma

a. is another name for tinea cruris
b. can be diagnosed with the aid of Wood's light
c. is a self-limiting condition
d. is caused by a corynebacterium
e. responds to griseofulvin therapy

For answers see over

Answers

A.3.16 a. T
        b. T
        c. F—The colour may be lost but retention of pigment is much commoner.
        d. F—A normal variant.
        e. F—This is the resting phase.

A.3.17 a. T—Frequently found in association with nickel.
        b. T—Especially by handling cement and tanned leather.
        c. T—Mercury-containing antiseptics are still available.
        d. F—Argyria, which results from exposure to silver, is not contact dermatitis.
        e. F

A.3.18 a. F—They are highly effective in giving short-term relief, but rebound worsening is usual when they are stopped.
        b. T—In less than 10% of cases is the onset before the age of 10.
        c. F—The arthropathy is seronegative.
        d. T
        e. F

A.3.19 a. T—The distinction is mainly based on the history.
        b. F—The typical central plug is never found in a BCC.
        c. F—No growth is to be expected after 3 months.
        d. T
        e. F—It resolves spontaneously if left.

A.3.20 a. F—But the groin is the commonest area affected.
        b. T—Coral pink fluorescence is characteristic.
        c. F—If untreated it will persist indefinitely.
        d. T
        e. F

Paper 4

Questions

Q.4.1 Tuberose sclerosis

a. is commoner in males
b. produces periungual fibromata
c. causes patchy hypopigmentation evident at birth
d. is always associated with epilepsy or mental deficiency or both
e. causes telangiectatic lesions of the face

Q.4.2 Long-term actinic damage to the skin may result in

a. elastoid degeneration
b. senile keratoses
c. senile comedones
d. decreased sebum secretion
e. senile purpura

Q.4.3 A livedo reticularis type of pattern on the skin

a. may occur in a physiological form in neonates
b. may indicate the presence of a vasculitis
c. can be induced by external heat
d. may be improved by the use of vasodilators
e. varies on a day-to-day basis

Q.4.4 Patients with acne vulgaris

a. are predisposed to develop rosacea in later life
b. may improve on a course of co-trimoxazole
c. are likely to be made worse by a course of corticosteroids
d. have a high sebum excretion rate
e. have an abnormal skin surface flora

Q.4.5 Antimalarials of the 4-aminoquinolone type (e.g. chloroquine)

a. may be beneficial in discoid lupus erythematosus
b. may be beneficial in psoriasis
c. can cause an irreversible retinopathy
d. may be helpful in rheumatoid arthritis
e. will improve rosacea

For answers see over

Answers

A.4.1   a. F—This condition is autosomal dominant.
          b. T—These occur during adult life.
          c. T—Best seen under Wood's light.
          d. F—There may be no evidence of CNS involvement.
          e. T—These are seen from the age of 2 onwards.

A.4.2   a. T
          b. T—Synonym is solar keratoses.
          c. T
          d. F—Decreased sebum secretion is a feature of old age but not directly linked to light exposure.
          e. F—Purpura is a feature of old age but not directly linked to light exposure.

A.4.3   a. T—Cutis marmorata.
          b. T—In this case it usually takes on an interrupted, broken distribution.
          c. T—Erythema ab igne.
          d. F
          e. F—It remains fairly static.

A.4.4   a. F—Despite the old name "acne rosacea", there is no connection between the two conditions.
          b. T
          c. F—It may well improve the inflammatory component.
          d. T
          e. F

A.4.5   a. T
          b. F—They often make it worse.
          c. T
          d. T
          e. F

Q.4.6 Pyoderma gangrenosum

a. is caused by synergistic infection with streptococci and staphylococci
b. requires surgical debridement
c. responds to systemic corticosteroids
d. may complicate ulcerative colitis
e. may complicate osteoarthritis

Q.4.7 Cutaneous lesions which may be associated with an endocrine abnormality include

a. epidermolysis bullosa
b. vitiligo
c. morphoea
d. necrobiosis lipoidica
e. neurofibromatosis

Q.4.8 Correct synonyms include

a. eczema and dermatitis
b. tuberose sclerosis and Bourneville's disease
c. toxic epidermal necrolysis and Lyell's disease
d. strawberry naevus and capillary haemangioma
e. senile keratosis and seborrhoeic keratosis

Q.4.9 A 60-year-old woman with multiple, smooth-surfaced, off-white asymptomatic plaques in the periorbital area might be suffering from

a. tuberose xanthomata
b. xanthelasmata
c. senile comedones
d. solar keratoses
e. syringomata

Q.4.10 Angio-oedema

a. may be linked with C_1 esterase inhibitor deficiency
b. may cause fatal obstruction of the airways
c. is also called urticaria pigmentosa
d. frequently has a nervous origin
e. will respond to antihistamines when idiopathic

For answers see over

Answers

A.4.6 a. F—It is a vasculitis not an infection.
      b. F
      c. T
      d. T—Usually indicates a very active phase of the disease.
      e. F—It may complicate *rheumatoid* arthritis.

A.4.7 a. F
      b. T—There is a slightly increased incidence to disorders giving tissue-specific autoantibodies, e.g. pernicious anaemia.
      c. F
      d. T—Diabetes is common.
      e. T—Phaeochromocytoma is a rare complication.

A.4.8 a. T—Dermatitis when not otherwise qualified (e.g. dermatitis herpetiformis) is the same as eczema.
      b. T—Also known as adenoma sebaceum.
      c. T
      d. F—Strawberry naevus = cavernous haemangioma; capillary haemangioma = naevus flammeus or port wine stain.
      e. F—Senile keratosis = solar keratosis; seborrhoeic keratosis = seborrhoeic wart.

A.4.9 a. F—Tuberose xanthomata do not occur on the face.
      b. T—Xanthelasmata are a common cause of such lesions.
      c. T—Senile comedones are frequently seen and are due to actinic damage.
      d. F
      e. T—Such lesions are often mistaken for xanthelasmata.

A.4.10 a. T—This is a rare familial type.
      b. T—But very rarely and usually only when caused by a severe allergy.
      c. F—It is also known as mastocytosis of the skin.
      d. F—The old name "angioneurotic oedema" has been dropped for this reason.
      e. T

Q.4.11 Alopecia areata

a. does not occur before puberty
b. gives slight scaling in the areas of hair loss
c. may cause slight pinkness in the bald areas
d. may occur in the beard area in men in the absence of scalp lesions
e. is a different disease from alopecia universalis

Q.4.12 Patients with atopic eczema have a greater than normal tendency to

a. develop allergic contact dermatitis
b. suffer from food allergy
c. react adversely to triple immunisation (diphtheria, tetanus, pertussis)
d. develop cutaneous pyogenic infections
e. suffer from herpes simplex

Q.4.13 An elderly man who has a gravitational ulcer with surrounding eczema might benefit from

a. Betnovate-C ointment applied daily
b. diuretic therapy to reduce the oedema
c. a supporting elastic bandage
d. povidine-iodine ointment to the ulcer
e. Lassar's paste applied round the ulcer

Q.4.14 Psoriasis

a. is present in about 0.2% of a Caucasian population
b. may demonstrate the isomorphic phenomenon
c. is associated with osteoarthritis
d. is associated with sub-total villous atrophy
e. may be precipitated by a viral sore throat

Q.4.15 Seborrhoeic warts

a. are caused by a human papilloma virus
b. may be spread venereally
c. arise from sebaceous glands
d. may be removed by curettage
e. respond to cryotherapy

For answers see over

Answers

A.4.11 a. F—It is quite common in children.
b. F—The areas show no epidermal changes.
c. T
d. T
e. F—The difference is believed to be one of degree.

A.4.12 a. F—There is a slightly reduced tendency to type 4 hypersensitivity.
b. T—Although this is not the cause of their eczema.
c. F—Smallpox immunisation is the only one associated with real problems.
d. T—Such infection is due to breaks in the skin surface barrier rather than any immunological cause.
e. F—Although the primary infection might be severe (Kaposi's varicelliform eruption).

A.4.13 a. F—This might help the eczema but would delay healing of the ulcer.
b. F—Diuretics do not clear gravitational oedema.
c. T
d. T—This is a useful antiseptic with a low capacity to sensitise.
e. T—This provides a useful protective to the surrounding skin.

A.4.14 a. F—The figure is about 2.0%.
b. T—Synonym is Köbner phenomenon.
c. F—Psoriasis is associated with seronegative arthritis of an atypical rheumatoid type or an ankylosing spondylitis.
d. F—Although slight mucosal changes have been reported.
e. F—Psoriasis may be precipitated by a streptococcal sore throat.

A.4.15 a. F
b. F—They are totally non-infectious.
c. F—Histologically they are basal cell papillomata.
d. T—Excision is never necessary.
e. T—Usually preferable to any form of surgery.

Q.4.16 A mole should be treated as malignant if

a. it shows the presence of coarse hairs
b. it is surrounded by a halo of vitiligo
c. it occurs as an enlarging nodule on a congenital giant bathing trunk naevus
d. it is still growing in a 30-year-old adult
e. it has bled on more than one occasion in an 8-year-old child

Q.4.17 Syphilis

a. of the primary type produces a painful chancre
b. of the secondary type typically affects the palms and soles
c. may produce condylomata accuminata in the perineum
d. ceases to be very infectious once the primary lesion has disappeared
e. may produce considerable scarring in the tertiary phase

Q.4.18 Hand-foot-and-mouth disease

a. is contracted from animals
b. is caused by a Coxsackie virus
c. causes marked debility
d. is commoner in children
e. resolves without treatment

Q.4.19 Scabies

a. is characteristically more itchy at night
b. will respond to treatment with benzoic acid compound ointment
c. nearly always involves the hands
d. may be non-irritating for the first 4 weeks
e. does not occur in the elderly

Q.4.20 Of leprosy it is true to state that

a. infection is transmitted most commonly by nasal discharge
b. tuberculoid leprosy is more rapidly progressive than lepromatous leprosy
c. hypopigmented anaesthetic patches are typical of tuberculoid leprosy
d. dapsone is the treatment of choice in lepromatous leprosy
e. lepromatous leprosy produces a leonine facies

For answers see over

Answers

A.4.16 a. F—This is a very sure sign of non-malignancy.
b. F—A Sutton's (halo) naevus is always benign.
c. T—The risk of malignancy is reputedly high.
d. T—Junctional activity usually ceases in the late teens.
e. F—Malignancy is exceptionally rare in childhood.

A.4.17 a. F—Chancres are typically painless.
b. T—This is very characteristic.
c. F—It may produce condylomata *lata*.
d. F—It remains highly infectious throughout the secondary phase.
e. T—Gummata are highly destructive.

A.4.18 a. F
b. T—Usually A16, but others have been implicated.
c. F—Debility is slight, especially in children.
d. T
e. T

A.4.19 a. T
b. F—It will respond to Whitfield's ointment, which is mildly fungicidal.
c. T
d. T—The irritation is due to an immunological response to the mite which takes some time to develop.
e. F—The prevalence is quite high in homes for the elderly.

A.4.20 a. T
b. F
c. T
d. F—Dapsone is cheap and effective, but rifampicin will render the condition non-infectious most rapidly.
e. T

Paper 5

Q.5.1 Skin disease in an otherwise healthy human may be caused by

a. *Tolypocladium inflatum*
b. *Microsporum canis*
c. *Trichophyton verrucosum*
d. *Pneumocystis carinii*
e. *Staphylococcus epidermidis*

Q.5.2 Premalignant lesions of the skin include

a. seborrhoeic keratoses
b. solar keratoses
c. parapsoriasis
d. histiocytoma
e. epidermal naevi

Q.5.3 Contact dermatitis is a not infrequent complication of the topical use of the antibiotic

a. chlortetracycline
b. mupirocin
c. framycetin
d. Fucidin
e. chloramphenicol

Q.5.4 Patchy depigmentation of the skin may be a feature of

a. pityriasis versicolor
b. adenoma sebaceum
c. lichen sclerosus et atrophicus
d. Addison's disease
e. morphoea

Q.5.5 Infection of the skin with *Staphylococcus aureus* might give rise to

a. cellulitis
b. furunculosis
c. scalded skin syndrome
d. erythema nodosum
e. pemphigus neonatorum

For answers see over

Answers

A.5.1   a. F—This is the organism from which cyclosporin is derived.
  b. T—This is a fungus of dogs and cats which can affect humans, particularly children.
  c. T—This fungus causes cattle ringworm, which can spread to man.
  d. F—A degree of immunosuppression. e.g. from AIDS, is essential.
  e. F—This is a normal skin commensal but it does have a predeliction for plastic, e.g. in IV lines and prosthetic valves.

A.5.2   a. F
  b. T—Squamous cell carcinomata may develop.
  c. T—Parapsoriasis may progress after many years to mycosis fungoides.
  d. F—Histiocytoma is a benign scar-like lesion (syn. dermatofibroma).
  e. T—Basal cell carcinomata may develop.

A.5.3   a. F
  b. F
  c. T—Framycetin cross reacts with neomycin.
  d. F
  e. T

A.5.4   a. T—On the light-exposed areas.
  b. T—Synonym is tuberose sclerosis. "Ash leaf" patches of depigmentation may be the first sign and are present at birth.
  c. T
  d. F—*Hyper*pigmentation is a feature of Addison's disease.
  e. T—Synonym is localised scleroderma.

A.5.5   a. F—Streptococci may give rise to cellulitis; staphylococci produce local abscesses.
  b. T
  c. T—But "staphylococcal scalded skin syndrome" only occurs in children.
  d. F
  e. T—A synonym for impetigo in the neonate.

Q.5.6   Dermatitis herpetiformis

a. has a similar distribution to chronic plaque psoriasis
b. is very itchy
c. clears rapidly on a gluten-free diet
d. is commoner in the elderly
e. is treated with low-dose systemic steroids

Q.5.7   Generalised pruritus may be a feature of

a. polycythaemia rubra vera
b. Hodgkin's disease
c. pityriasis rosea
d. haemolytic jaundice
e. diabetes mellitus

Q.5.8   Acne vulgaris

a. occurs only in the teens and early twenties
b. is more severe in patients with poor personal hygiene
c. responds to systemic erythromycin
d. may be treated with topical steroid creams
e. is worse when the sebum excretion rate is high

Q.5.9   Cryotherapy is suitable treatment for

a. seborrhoeic keratoses
b. warty naevi
c. basal cell carcinomata
d. solar keratoses
e. periungual viral warts

Q.5.10   Chemicals effective as screening agents against UVB include

a. mexenone
b. para-aminobenzoic acid
c. benzydamine
d. titanium dioxide
e. 1% hydrocortisone cream

For answers see over

Answers

A.5.6 a. T—It occurs on the elbows and knees and in the sacral area particularly.
        b. T—The main symptom is itchiness.
        c. F—Any improvement is very slow indeed.
        d. F—Individuals may be affected at any age from childhood onwards.
        e. F—Dapsone is the treatment of choice.

A.5.7 a. T—Particularly after bathing.
        b. T
        c. T
        d. F—It is a feature of obstructive jaundice.
        e. F—Although it is given as a cause in older textbooks.

A.5.8 a. F—It may persist throughout adult life.
        b. F—Blackheads are not due to dirt.
        c. T
        d. F—Although the inflammation will be suppressed.
        e. T—But this is not the only factor.

A.5.9 a. T
        b. F—They are unresponsive.
        c. F—The response is unreliable.
        d. T
        e. F—Cryotherapy is effective, but the risk of damage to the nail is high.

A.5.10 a. T—Uvistat is one example.
        b. T—Spectraban 15 is one example.
        c. F—This is a topical non-steroid anti-inflammatory drug (proprietary name Difflam).
        d. T—This preparation is opaque and therefore highly effective.
        e. F—Although anti-inflammatory after the event it has no screening properties.

Q.5.11 The following are features of systemic sclerosis:

a. Dysphagia
b. Conjunctivitis sicca
c. Soft tissue calcification
d. Perforated nasal septum
e. Pulmonary diffusion defect

Q.5.12 The Köbner phenomenon is seen in

a. pityriasis rosea
b. viral warts
c. parapsoriasis
d. molluscum contagiosum
e. herpes zoster

Q.5.13 Irritation in the vulval area in the absence of cutaneous lesions elsewhere may be due to

a. contact dermatitis
b scabies
c. idiopathic pruritus vulvae
d. lichen sclerosus et atrophicus
e. psoriasis

Q.5.14 Lichen planus

a. may involve mucous membranes
b. may cause hair loss
c. is rarely itchy
d. can result from drugs
e. responds to topical therapy with 1% hydrocortisone

Q.5.15 Excessive growth of hair

a. is known as "hirsutism" only when it has a male distribution in the female
b. is a feature of the Stein–Leventhal syndrome
c. may be seen in epileptics as a result of phenobarbitone therapy
d. is sometimes seen in Cushing's disease
e. is a feature of systemic lupus erythematosus

For answers see over

Answers

A.5.11 a. T—Often an early symptom.
  b. T—As part of Sjögren's syndrome.
  c. T—As part of the CRST syndrome (calcinosis cutis, Raynaud's phenomenon, sclerodactyly, telangiectasis).
  d. F
  e. T

A.5.12 a. F
  b. T—Especially the "plane" type.
  c. F—Unlike true psoriasis.
  d. F
  e. F

A.5.13 a. T
  b. F—Scabies can be ruled out in the absence of lesions elsewhere.
  c. T—Idiopathic pruritus vulvae is the commonest cause.
  d. T
  e. T—Psoriasis may affect just one area.

A.5.14 a. T—Both oral and anal mucous membranes may be affected.
  b. T—Hair loss can occur in the uncommon scalp form known as lichen planopilaris.
  c. F—Severe irritation is usual.
  d. T—Particularly gold and antimalarials.
  e. F—Strong topical or systemic steroids are required.

A.5.15 a. T—Otherwise it it called hypertrichosis.
  b. T
  c. F—It may be caused by phenytoin.
  d. T
  e. F

Q.5.16 Hair loss with scarring may be found in

a. lichen planus
b. seborrhoeic dermatitis
c. alopecia areata
d. discoid lupus erythematosus
e. herpes zoster

Q.5.17 Deformity of the nails may be found in association with

a. periungual mucoid cysts
b. chronic paronychia
c. alopecia areata
d. pemphigoid
e. parapsoriasis

Q.5.18 Infantile seborrhoeic dermatitis

a. is itchy
b. can look like psoriasis
c. is caused by ammoniacal irritation in the napkin area
d. is a cause of failure to thrive
e. is a juvenile form of adult seborrhoeic dermatitis

Q.5.19 Risk factors of developing cutaneous malignancy include

a. ultraviolet light exposure
b. renal transplantation
c. tar therapy for psoriasis
d. xeroderma pigmentosum
e. epidermolysis bullosa

Q.5.20 Lavatory seats

a. are a source of scabies
b. may cause contact dermatitis
c. may harbour poisonous spiders
d. can transmit pubic lice
e. are rare in Asia

For answers see over

Answers

A.5.16 a. T—It is a rare complication of lichen planus of the scalp.
b. F—Although slight hair loss is common.
c. F—This is a cause of non-scarring alopecia.
d. T—Typically it occurs with keratinous plugging of the follicles.
e. T

A.5.17 a. T—A concave groove is frequent.
b. T
c. T
d. F
e. F

A.5.18 a. F—It gives no symptoms.
b. T—It is thought by some to be a form of psoriasis.
c. F—Although irritation of the skin in the area will make it worse.
d. F—It rarely causes any upset to the child.
e. F—The two conditions are unrelated.

A.5.19 a. T—The fairer the skin the higher the risk.
b. T—Due to immunosuppressant therapy.
c. F—Any effect is thought to be negligible.
d. T—A classic, if incredibly rare, defect in the ability to repair UV-damaged DNA.
e. T—Of the autosomal recessive dystrophic type; a common cause of death.

A.5.20 a. F—Skin-to-skin contact is necessary.
b. T—Particularly the wooden variety.
c. T—In Australia, for example.
d. F—Pubic-to-pubic contact is the usual method of transmission.
e. T

Paper 6

Q.6.1 Conditions which may be evident at birth include

    a. neonatal acne
    b. cavernous haemangiomata
    c. small pigmented naevi
    d. ichthyosis
    e. incontinentia pigmenti

Q.6.2 Eccrine sweat glands

    a. are most numerous on the palms and soles
    b. function poorly in the first few weeks of life
    c. open onto the pilosebaceous unit
    d. are blocked in prickly heat
    e. may be deficient in ichthyosis vulgaris

Q.6.3 Nailfold telangiectasia is a feature of

    a. rheumatoid arthritis
    b. Raynaud's phenomenon
    c. dermatomyositis
    d. discoid lupus erythematosus
    e. erythrodermic psoriasis

Q.6.4 Rosacea

    a. is commoner in women
    b. causes a "butterfly" eruption on the face
    c. spreads onto the scalp when severe
    d. starts at puberty in 10% of cases
    e. responds to therapy with metronidazole

Q.6.5 Explanation and reassurance is usually all that is required in the management of

    a. alopecia areata
    b. acne vulgaris
    c. minimal psoriasis confined to the knees and elbows
    d. keratoacanthoma
    e. pityriasis rosea

For answers see over

Answers

A.6.1 a. F—The condition appears during the first few months of life.
b. F—The lesions start appearing during the first few days of life.
c. F—Although the unusual "giant" or "bathing trunk" type are evident at birth.
d. T—The condition may be unduly severe at birth and may present as a "collodion baby".
e. T—This is a rare disorder restricted to girls. Firm intact blisters may be seen.

A.6.2 a. T
b. T
c. F
d. T
e. F—Although they are deficient in some other forms of ichthyosis.

A.6.3 a. F
b. T—Whatever the cause.
c. T
d. T
e. F

A.6.4 a. T—Although the difference in incidence between the sexes is slight.
b. F—Affects both cheeks separately.
c. T—Characteristically the lesions stop at the hair margin.
d. F—It is a disease of middle life.
e. T

A.6.5 a. T—In the vast majority of cases the condition resolves and treatment is unsatisfactory.
b. F—Active treatment is nearly always helpful.
c. T—Total eradication of all psoriatic plaques is often not possible.
d. F—Although it is a lesion which resolves spontaneously, scarring will result if it is left untreated.
e. T—Except in the occasional case where irritation is a problem.

Q.6.6   Necrobiosis lipoidica

a. is most commonly located on the shins
b. causes telangiectasia and dermal thickening
c. may ulcerate
d. is never found in the absence of diabetes
e. improves with good control of the diabetes

Q.6.7   Dermatomyositis

a. causes a distal myopathy
b. may result in muscle calcification in children
c. is invariably fatal
d. causes a rise in the serum creatine phosphokinase
e. may be associated with internal malignancy

Q.6.8   Cheilitis

a. may be a manifestation of atopic eczema in children
b. of the angular type is more common in people with dentures
c. may be produced by retinoids
d. is frequently premalignant
e. may result from actinic damage

Q.6.9   Hidradenitis suppurativa

a. is the correct name for prickly heat
b. is a disorder of apocrine glands
c. affects mainly the axillae and groins
d. is characterised by recurrent abscesses infected with *Staphylococcus aureus*
e. responds to short (7-day) courses of antibiotics

Q.6.10   Stevens–Johnson syndrome

a. is a *forme fruste* of Behçet's disease
b. may be caused by drugs
c. may follow a viral infection
d. affects the mouth but not the genitalia
e. remits spontaneously

For answers see over

Answers

A.6.6
a. T—But it can occur on other areas.
b. F—Telangiectasia and dermal atrophy are characteristic.
c. T
d. F—In about 50% of cases there is no evidence of diabetes mellitus.
e. F—Sadly it does not.

A.6.7
a. F—It causes a proximal myopathy.
b. T—This may cause permanent disability.
c. F—But it may cause death.
d. T—This is an important indicator of disease activity.
e. T—But only in adults is this association found.

A.6.8
a. T—Licking the slightly rough lips becomes a habit.
b. T—Slight pooling of saliva and candidiasis are responsible.
c. T—It is the commonest side effect.
d. F—It is premalignant only when light exposure is the cause.
e. T

A.6.9
a. F
b. T
c. T
d. F—Abscesses are the main problem, but recognised pathogens are not grown from them.
e. F—It is an intractable condition which responds poorly to antibiotics.

A.6.10
a. F—It is a form of erythema multiforme affecting mainly the mucosae.
b. T—But viral infections are a commoner cause.
c. T—Especially herpes simplex.
d. F—Both are affected, but the mouth is involved more frequently.
e. T—Treatment is symptomatic only.

Q.6.11 Involvement of the nails is a feature of

a. thyrotoxicosis
b. systemic sclerosis
c. lichen planus
d. alopecia areata
e. necrobiosis lipoidica

Q.6.12 Atopic eczema is

a. commoner in boys
b. inherited as a simple Mendelian dominant
c. associated with an increased risk of infection
d. a cause of white dermographism
e. treatable with topical antihistamines

Q.6.13 Psoriasis

a. often affects the sacral area
b. involves the oral mucosa on rare occasions
c. in the guttate form does not involve the scalp
d. may cover the whole skin surface
e. may affect the nails in the absence of lesions elsewhere

Q.6.14 Premalignant conditions of the skin include

a. poikiloderma vasculare atrophicans
b. Hutchinson's freckle
c. oral leukoplakia
d. sebaceous naevus
e. lichen sclerosus et atrophicus

Q.6.15 Malignant melanoma

a. is rare in blacks
b. is decreasing in frequency because of better diagnostic techniques
c. is a radiosensitive tumour
d. carries a universally poor prognosis
e. may be totally non-pigmented

For answers see over

Answers

A.6.11 a. F
      b. T—It is due to the poor peripheral circulation.
      c. T
      d. T—Occasionally the nails are the sole site of the disorder.
      e. F

A.6.12 a. F—The sex incidence is equal.
      b. F—The mode of inheritance is not clear.
      c. T—It is due to colonisation of the broken skin.
      d. T—But not the only one.
      e. F—Nothing should be treated with topical antihistamines.

A.6.13 a. T—Almost as commonly as it affects the elbows and knees.
      b. T—But only very rarely.
      c. F—Scalp lesions can help in differentiating it from other conditions, e.g. pityriasis rosea.
      d. T—It is a frequent cause of erythroderma.
      e. T

A.6.14 a. T—After many years this condition may develop into mycosis fungoides, a T cell lymphoma of the skin.
      b. T—Synonym is lentigo maligna, a slowly growing malignant melanoma.
      c. T—Squamous cell carcinoma may develop.
      d. T—Basal cell carcinoma may develop.
      e. F—But this condition is often confused with vulval leukoplakia.

A.6.15 a. T—But it does occur.
      b. F—There is a steady worldwide increase.
      c. F—Less than 10% of cases will show any response.
      d. F—Some forms, e.g. lentigo maligna melanoma, carry a very good prognosis.
      e. T—Amelanotic melanoma is non-pigmented.

Q.6.16 Of shingles (herpes zoster) it is true to state that

a. it may be associated with a malignant lymphoma
b. neuralgia is a frequent complication in the young
c. topical acyclovir is useful if started early in an attack
d. in patients with atopic eczema it may produce Kaposi's varicelliform eruption
e. pain never precedes the development of vesicles

Q.6.17 A sore throat might precede

a. a morbilliform eruption caused by ampicillin administration
b. hot painful nodules on the lower limb
c. erythema marginatum
d. an attack of lichen planus
e. pityriasis rosea

Q.6.18 Tinea capitis

a. occurs only in children
b. may be contracted from animals
c. does not respond to griseofulvin
d. fluoresces pink with Wood's light
e. causes inflammation of the scalp as well as hair loss

Q.6.19 Regarding childhood exanthemata:

a. The eruption of chickenpox follows 3 days of malaise
b. Primary herpes simplex is likely to be more severe in children with atopic eczema
c. Rubella is more severe in mentally retarded children
d. Measles may cause an encephalitis
e. Chickenpox can be most rapidly diagnosed by electron microscopy of blister fluid

Q.6.20 Occlusive support bandaging of the leg is helpful in the management of

a. traumatic damage to the skin
b. lichen simplex (neurodermatitis)
c. ischaemic ulceration
d. diabetic ulceration
e. erythema nodosum

For answers see over

Answers

A.6.16 a. T—In this case a chickenpox-like eruption may occur as well.

        b. F—Neuralgia is rare in the young but its incidence increases with age.

        c. T—But the key to success is starting treatment early enough.

        d. F—This condition is due to herpes simplex.

        e. F—Pain may be the initial complaint.

A.6.17 a. T—Glandular fever.

        b. T—Erythema nodosum.

        c. T—The classic eruption of rheumatic fever.

        d. F

        e. F

A.6.18 a. T

        b. T—Kittens and puppies are particular sources of infection (*Microsporum canis*).

        c. F

        d. F—The fluorescence has a greeny-yellow colour.

        e. T—This is one of the characteristic features.

A.6.19 a. T—But this general malaise may be slight in young children.

        b. T—It may cause Kaposi's varicelliform eruption.

        c. F

        d. T

        e. T—But a distinction from herpes simplex cannot be made.

A.6.20 a. T—Treat as for gravitational ulceration.

        b. T—Protection from further damage from scratching is helpful.

        c. F—Bandaging will further impair the circulation.

        d. F—A neuropathic limb may be traumatised by an elastic bandage.

        e. T—It helps to relieve pain.

Paper 7

Q.7.1 The *minority* of basal cell carcinomata show

a. hyperkeratosis
b. cystic degeneration
c. telangiectasia
d. pigmentation
e. scarring

Q.7.2 A high capacity to produce contact dermatitis is shown by

a. DMSO (dimethyl sulphoxide)
b. terpenes
c. colophony
d. polyvinyl chloride
e. epoxy resins

Q.7.3 A course of systemic steroids is suitable treatment for

a. pemphigus neonatorum
b. systemic sclerosis
c. dermatomyositis
d. pemphigoid
e. urticaria

Q.7.4 Tinea capitis

a. responds to treatment with topical antifungals
b. may cause permanent alopecia
c. always fluoresces under Wood's light
d. occurs almost exclusively in children
e. can be contracted from kittens

Q.7.5 Patchy hypopigmentation may be a feature of

a. lichen sclerosus et atrophicus
b. tuberose sclerosis
c. pityriasis rosea
d. morphoea
e. facial eczema

For answers see over

Answers

A.7.1 a. F—Hyperkeratosis is not a feature of basal cell carcinomata.
    b. T—This may be quite marked.
    c. F—Telangiectasia is a feature of almost all basal cell carcinomata.
    d. T—Occasionally the pigmentation is severe enough to mimic a melanoma.
    e. T—Scarring is a feature of a particularly slow growing type of basal cell carcinoma.

A.7.2 a. F—This useful solvent aids penetration of topical medicaments.
    b. T—These are members of a large group of plant extracts which are used in perfumes etc.
    c. T—This resin, another plant extract, is the sensitiser in sticking plasters.
    d. F—PVC is almost inert.
    e. T—Particularly in the uncured state.

A.7.3 a. F—This condition is a staphylococcal infection of the newborn.
    b. F—Systemic sclerosis is unresponsive.
    c. T
    d. T—The dose may have to be high.
    e. F—Antihistamines are preferable.

A.7.4 a. F—Systemic griseofulvin is required.
    b. T—Severe untreated tinea capitis may scar.
    c. F—It usually does, but this is dependent on the organism.
    d. T
    e. T—And puppies, usually due to *Microsporum canis*.

A.7.5 a. T
    b. T—And it may be present at birth.
    c. F—It is a feature of pityriasis versicolor.
    d. T
    e. T—Pityriasis alba is the mildest form.

Q.7.6 In pemphigoid

a. blisters arise on otherwise normal skin
b. direct immunofluorescence shows immunoglobulin deposition at the epidermo-dermal junction
c. oral ulceration is often the presenting feature
d. the 45–65 age group is most commonly affected
e. ultimate remission is usual

Q.7.7 Keratin is

a. normally orthokeratotic
b. parakeratotic at wound edges
c. parakeratotic in psoriasis
d. is parakeratotic when the granular layer is thickened
e. rich in disulphide bonds

Q.7.8 Miliaria

a. may be seen in neonates
b. disappears without treatment in a few weeks
c. may produce superficial vesicles
d. is spread by anopheles mosquitos
e. is common in people living in the tropics

Q.7.9 Topical preparations which can be bought without prescription in the UK include

a. local anaesthetics
b. antihistamines
c. 2.5% hydrocortisone
d. some antibiotics
e. imidazole antifungals

Q.7.10 Skin conditions associated with diabetes include

a. furunculosis
b. pityriasis versicolor
c. necrobiosis lipoidica
d. pyoderma gangrenosum
e. balanitis

For answers see over

Answers

A.7.6 a. F—The skin usually shows sheets of erythema before the blisters appear.
b. T
c. F—Pemphig*us* starts in this way.
d. F—Pemphigus again; usual age for pemphigoid is 70+ (mostly over 80).
e. T—Most patients can be weaned off treatment.

A.7.7 a. T—The nuclei are lost.
b. T—The nuclei are retained due to rapid growth.
c. T—A very characteristic feature of the histology.
d. F—It is in the granular layer that the nuclei are lost in normal keratin.
e. T

A.7.8 a. T—It is usually caused by wearing too many clothes.
b. T—Even if high temperatures continue.
c. T—In miliaria crystallina superficial vesicles are produced.
d. F
e. F—Visitors to the tropics get it.

A.7.9 a. T
b. T
c. F—The maximum concentration available without prescription is 1%.
d. F
e. T

A.7.10 a. T—The severity, if not the frequency, is increased.
b. F
c. T—This condition classically produces atrophic, waxy telangiectatic lesions on the shins.
d. F
e. T—This is due to candidiasis.

Q.7.11   It is true to state that

a. allergic contact dermatitis is mediated by lymphocytes
b. atopic eczema is associated with high circulating levels of IgE
c the effector chemical in eccrine sweat glands is adrenaline
d. percutaneous absorption is enhanced by hydration of the horny layer
e. acne pustules are caused by *Staphylococcus pyogenes*

Q.7.12   Granuloma annulare

a. is characterised by scaling erythematous annular lesions
b. is commoner in children
c. affects the hands and feet most frequently
d. is itchy
e. shows a strong association with diabetes

Q.7.13   Oral ulcers are an occasional feature of

a. pemphigus vulgaris
b. erythema multiforme
c. primary herpes simplex infection
d. methotrexate toxicity
e. iron deficiency

Q.7.14   Psychogenic factors are believed to play at least some part in

a. hyperhidrosis of the palms
b. acné excoriée
c. sycosis barbae
d. dermatitis artefacta
e. urticaria

Q.7.15   Benign pigmented cellular naevi

a. are most common in Caucasians
b. may develop a halo of vitiligo and disappear spontaneously
c. show junctional activity throughout life
d. are confined to the epidermis
e. should be excised prophylactically to prevent malignancy occurring

For answers see over

Answers

A.7.11 a. T—A type IV cell-mediated immune response.
      b. T—Usually higher than in atopics with asthma or rhinitis.
      c. F—The nerves are cholinergic sympathetic.
      d. T—Hence the use of steroids under polythene occlusion in refractory dermatoses.
      e. F—They contain *Propionibacterium acnes,* and the inflammatory response is due to the breakdown of neutral lipids into fatty acids.

A.7.12 a. F—It is characterised by pale dermal nodules in an annular distribution.
      b. T
      c. T
      d. F—It is asymptomatic apart from the appearance.
      e. F—Any link is very tenuous.

A.7.13 a. F—They are an almost universal feature of pemphigus vulgaris.
      b. T—The Stevens–Johnson syndrome.
      c. T—This is the usual presentation in neonates but not in older age groups.
      d. T
      e. F—Stomatitis is a feature of iron deficiency, but not with ulceration.

A.7.14 a. T—Stress is the main cause.
      b. T—Squeezing facial spots becomes compulsive.
      c. F—This is folliculitis of the beard.
      d. T—Self-inflicted lesions are the hallmark.
      e. F

A.7.15 a. T
      b. T—So-called Sutton's or halo naevus.
      c. F—Junctional activity in a mole in an adult should be regarded as a sign of malignant potential.
      d. F—They are mainly dermal.
      e. F

Q.7.16 Atopic eczema

a. as a manifestation of the atopic state is about half as common as asthma
b. may be present in the absence of irritation
c. is due to the same range of allergens as asthma
d. responds well to treatment with non-sedating antihistamines
e. often affects the face in young infants

Q.7.17 A fit young adult complains of an extremely tender solitary nodule of 2–3 mm diameter which examination reveals is entirely within the skin. Possible diagnoses include

a. Kaposi's sarcoma
b. leiomyoma
c. glomus tumour
d. blue naevus
e. keratoacanthoma

Q.7.18 The following tumours have no malignant potential:

a. Cutaneous viral warts
b. Seborrhoeic keratoses
c. Dermatofibromata
d. Hutchinson's lentigo
e. Keratoacanthoma

Q.7.19 The cutaneous manifestations of AIDS include

a. a rubella-like eruption
b. seborrhoeic dermatitis
c. Kaposi's varicelliform eruption
d. malignant angiosarcomata
e. dematophyte infections

Q.7.20 Scabies

a. can occur in the absence of itching
b. does not affect the face in adults
c. does not occur in infants less than 3 months old
d. shows an increased prevalence in institutionalised patients
e. rarely affects the penis

For answers see over

Answers

A.7.16 a. F—The frequency is about equal.
      b. F—Itching is the hallmark.
      c. F—It is difficult to prove that allergies play a part at all.
      d. F—Any benefit from antihistamines is probably only due to sedation.
      e. T—Initially the face may be the worst affected area.

A.7.17 a. F—This tumour is neither solitary nor painful.
      b. T
      c. T—This is the most exquisitely tender of all skin tumours.
      d. F
      e. F

A.7.18 a. T—But genital warts and cervical cancer have been linked.
      b. T
      c. T
      d. F—A malignant melanoma may eventually arise.
      e. T—But be sure of the diagnosis: A squamous cell carcinoma may look very similar.

A.7.19 a. T—This is found in the early stages.
      b. T
      c. F—Kaposi's sarcoma is a characteristic manifestation.
      d. T—Synonymous with Kaposi's sarcomata.
      e. T—These are often intractable.

A.7.20 a. T—In the early stages and in the immunocompromised.
      b. T—But the face is affected in young infants and in "Norwegian" scabies.
      c. F—It is a well-recognised cause of an itchy eruption at this age.
      d. T—It is spread by hand holding.
      e. F—It commonly does.

Paper 8

Q.8.1 **Blistering of the skin may be a prominent feature of**

a. burns
b. secondary syphilis
c. herpes gestationis
d. toxic epidermal necrolysis
e. pityriasis rosea

Q.8.2 **Generalised pruritus may be caused by**

a. low serum iron
b. cirrhosis of the liver
c. lymphoma
d. secondary syphilis
e. pregnancy

Q.8.3 **Gravitational (venous) ulcers**

a. may follow a previous fracture in the limb
b. deteriorate when contaminated with coliform organisms
c. are painful in most sufferers
d. are commoner in men
e. are often the result of varicose veins

Q.8.4 **Sebaceous glands are**

a. stimulated by oestrogens
b. innervated by cholinergic sympathetic nerves
c. holocrine glands
d. absent on the soles of the feet
e. present on the buccal mucosa

Q.8.5 **It is appropriate to treat**

a. psoriasis with 5% dithranol
b. dermatitis herpetiformis with co-trimoxazole
c. genital warts with 25% podophyllin in liquid paraffin
d. pemphigus with oral prednisolone
e. solar keratoses with 5% fluorouracil topically

For answers see over

Answers

A.8.1 a. T
  b. F
  c. T—This is an unusual but serious eruption of pregnancy which resembles pemphigoid.
  d. T—This is often severe and extensive.
  e. F

A.8.2 a. T—But rarely.
  b. T—Particularly primary biliary cirrhosis.
  c. T
  d. F—Typically, secondary syphilis is asymptomatic.
  e. T

A.8.3 a. T—This is the commonest cause in men.
  b. F—These organisms are almost universally present and seem to cause few problems.
  c. F—Pain is unusual in the absence of complications.
  d. F—They are commoner in women.
  e. F—Superficial varices are irrelevant or secondary.

A.8.4 a. F—They are stimulated by androgens and suppressed by oestrogens.
  b. F—This is the innvervation of eccrine sweat glands.
  c. T—The whole cell forms the secretion.
  d. T
  e. T—So-called Fordyce's spots.

A.8.5 a. F—The concentration is too high.
  b. F—Dapsone is the treatment of choice.
  c. T—A single application is often enough.
  d. T—High (100 mg +) doses are often required.
  e. T—This is a useful topical cytotoxic.

Q.8.6 An ulcer on the lower leg may be a feature of

a. rheumatoid arthritis
b. sickle cell anaemia
c. past poliomyelitis
d. previous fracture
e. superficial varicosities

Q.8.7 The cutaneous lesions of scurvy

a. resolve steadily after about 1 month of therapy
b. include purpura
c. are usually most marked on the lower legs
d. may be overshadowed by depression
e. include the breakdown of old scars

Q.8.8 A fishmonger with pain, redness and swelling around the nailfolds of the right thumb and index finger of 4 months' duration might be suffering from

a. herpes simplex paronychia
b. erysipeloid
c. candida paronychia
d. a condition which might benefit from a change of employment
e. acrodermatitis continua

Q.8.9 A lichenoid eruption can be induced by

a. the use of cytotoxic drugs
b. graft versus host disease
c. contact with colour photograph developer
d. myocrisin therapy for rheumatoid arthritis
e. antimalarials

Q.8.10 It is true to state that

a. pemphigoid is commonest in the over 80 age group
b. pityriasis rosea can be distinguished from secondary syphilis by the presence of palmar lesions in the former
c. Kaposi's sarcoma is rare in HIV-negative patients
d. surgical drainage is the treatment of choice for acne cysts
e. viral warts of the cervix uteri may be premalignant

For answers see over

Answers

A.8.6 a. T—The ulceration in rheumatoid arthritis may have several different causes.
   b. T—Infarcts occur in many organs, including the skin.
   c. F—Sensory impairment is necessary for neuropathic ulcers to develop.
   d. T—As a result of deep venous thrombosis.
   e. F—Damage to deep veins is required.

A.8.7 a. F—The response is extremely rapid once replacement therapy is started.
   b. T—Purpura is a hallmark of the disease.
   c. T
   d. T
   e. T

A.8.8 a. F—The history is too long.
   b. T—Usually this condition is acute but it may be chronic.
   c. T—The most likely diagnosis.
   d. T—Causes (b) and (c) are occupational, and cold, wet conditions are contributory.
   e. T—An unusual and chronic form of psoriasis.

A.8.9 a. F
   b. T—In the subacute stage.
   c. T
   d. T
   e. T

A.8.10 a. T
   b. F—It is the other way round: Palmar lesions are present in secondary syphilis.
   c. T
   d. F—Marked scarring often results.
   e. T

Q.8.11 **Scaling is a prominent feature of**

a. lichen sclerosus et atrophicus
b. morphoea
c. secondary syphilis
d. keratoderma blenorrhagica
e. granuloma annulare

Q.8.12 **Regarding the case of a 20-year-old woman who complains of excessive facial and body hair:**

a. her ethnic origins are irrelevant
b. a virilising adrenal tumour is a possibility
c. a history of weight gain and amenorrhoea may be relevant
d. extensive investigations are likely to be unrewarding if her periods are normal
e. testicular feminisation is a possibility

Q.8.13 **In a 12-year-old girl with extensive impetigo of her face**

a topical hydrocortisone is useful to settle the inflammation
b. associated infection with *Sarcoptes scabiei* is not uncommon
c. topical treatment with a tetracycline ointment is rapidly effective
d. systemic penicillin is effective treatment
e. she should be kept home from school

Q.8.14 **Hairs**

a. of the lanugo type are found in the fetus
b. of the terminal type are found only in old age
c. grow more strongly after shaving
d. may change from the vellus to terminal during life
e. grow continuously except when interrupted by illness (telogen effluvium)

Q.8.15 **An acute weeping eczema can be treated with**

a. corticosteroid ointments
b. coal tar paste
c. dithranol cream
d. local anaesthetics
e. shake lotions and compresses

For answers see over

Answers

A.8.11 a. T
          b. F
          c. T
          d. T
          e. F

A.8.12 a. F—There is a marked difference in the amount of body hair between different races, with the most hirsute being from the Indian subcontinent.
          b. T—There are always other signs of androgenisation.
          c. T—Such a history would assist a diagnosis of polycystic ovaries.
          d. T—Hormonal abnormalities are usually reflected first in an alteration of the menses.
          e. F—This is a condition where there is a total lack of response to androgens.

A.8.13 a. F
          b. F—Scabies is often secondarily infected but does not affect the face.
          c. T—Effective against both staphylococci and streptococci.
          d. F—Penicillin and its derivatives systemically administered are slow to reach the skin surface in therapeutic amounts.
          e. T—The condition is highly contagious.

A.8.14 a. T
          b. F—These are the normal coarse hairs of the scalp.
          c. F—This is a popular myth.
          d. T—For example, beard and body hair undergo this change.
          e. F—They grow cyclically.

A.8.15 a. F—But cream preparations can be used.
          b. F—Neither the tar nor the paste are suitable.
          c. F—This is the specific treatment for psoriasis.
          d. F
          e. T—The treatment of choice.

Q.8.16 **The individual lesions of psoriasis characteristically show**

a. an ill-defined edge
b. telangiectasia
c. thick adherent scale when occurring in the flexures
d. accentuation of the dermal papillae histologically
e. a lymphocytic infiltrate histologically

Q.8.17 **Malignant melanoma**

a. is more serious if the depth is greater than 0.72 mm
b. is less serious if it arises in a lentigo maligna
c. may arise from a deeply pigmented seborrhoeic wart
d. should always be treated surgically by removal of the primary together with the draining lymph nodes
e. will respond to cytotoxic therapy in about 30% of cases

Q.8.18 **Totally benign lesions which may affect the face include**

a. milia
b. solar keratoses
c. epidermal naevi
d. plane warts
e. capillary angiomata

Q.8.19 **Streptococcal tonsillitis may be implicated in the development of**

a. scalded skin syndrome in children
b. Henoch–Schönlein purpura
c. papular urticaria
d. erythema nodosum
e. pityriasis rosea

Q.8.20 **Pityriasis versicolor**

a. causes pale areas on light-exposed skin
b. is the cause of dandruff when it affects the scalp
c. responds to selenium-sulphide-containing preparations
d. starts with a herald patch
e. is commoner in humid climates

For answers see over

Answers

A.8.16 a. F—A well-defined edge is almost universal.
        b. F
        c. F—Flexural lesions usually do not scale.
        d. T
        e. F—Polymorphonuclear leucocytes are most prominent in the infiltrate.

A.8.17 a. T
        b. T
        c. F
        d. F—Only local removal is required, unless the lymph nodes are clinically involved.
        e. F—The response to any combination of cytotoxics is poor.

A.8.18 a. T
        b. F—Occasionally solar keratoses progress to squamous cell carcinomata.
        c. F—These may progress to basal cell carcinomata.
        d. T
        e. T—These may enlarge and produce nodules but they do not become malignant.

A.8.19 a. F—Staphylococci are the cause.
        b. T—Although not in every case.
        c. F—This is a euphemism for insect bites.
        d. T
        e. F

A.8.20 a. T—And light-brown ones on covered skin.
        b. F—Pityriasis capitis is the synonym for dandruff. Pityriasis versicolor does not affect the scalp.
        c. T—An example is Selsun shampoo.
        d. F—This is characteristic of pityriasis *rosea*.
        e. T

Paper 9

Q.9.1 **Viral warts**

    a. are all due to the same type of human papilloma virus
    b. may occasionally affect the larynx
    c. may be a sign of sexual abuse when present on the genitalia of children
    d. may be treated with a daily application of 25% podophyllin in liquid paraffin when present on the genitalia of adults
    e. will regress spontaneously in normal children

Q.9.2 **Sebaceous cysts**

    a. contain altered sebum
    b. are particularly common on the scalp
    c. are often telangiectatic
    d. should not be diagnosed in the absence of a punctum
    e. are localised to the epidermis

Q.9.3 **Blistering in the skin of a neonate might be due to**

    a. scabies
    b. seborrhoeic dermatitis
    c. epidermolysis bullosa
    d. impetigo
    e. atopic eczema

Q.9.4 **Light sensitivity may be a feature of**

    a. discoid lupus erythematosus
    b. dermatomyositis
    c. acute intermittent porphyria
    d. tetracycline therapy
    e. guttate psoriasis

Q.9.5 **Penile ulcers may result from**

    a. gonorrhoea
    b. Stevens–Johnson syndrome
    c. secondary syphilis
    d. severe aphthosis
    e. herpes simplex infection

For answers see over

Answers

A.9.1   a. F—There are many closely related types of papilloma virus which produce slightly different lesions clinically.
b. T—Usually in association with warts on the tongue.
c. T
d. F—The preparation is suitable, but one treatment is all that is required, repeated at 3-week intervals if necessary.
e. T

A.9.2   a. F—They are keratin cysts.
b. T
c. T
d. F—Although typical, a punctum is often not visible.
e. F—They are dermal, even though they arise from the epidermis.

A.9.3   a. F—Scabies does produce blisters, but these take time to develop.
b. F—Seborrhoeic dermatitis does not blister.
c. T
d. T—Synonym is pemphigus neonatorum.
e. F

A.9.4   a. T
b. F
c. F—This is the only abnormality of porphyrin metabolism which does not show light sensitivity
d. T—Particularly demethylchlortetracycline and doxycycline.
e. T—Any patient with erupting psoriasis, e.g. showing the Köbner phenomenon, may react adversely.

A.9.5   a. F
b. T
c. F
d. T
e. T

Q.9.6   Comedones contain significant quantities of

a. dried sebum
b. extraneous dirt
c. keratin
d. *Propionibacterium acnes*
e. melanin

Q.9.7   Erysipelas

a. is also called erysipeloid
b. is a form of cellulitis
c. is caused by malnutrition
d. may be recurrent
e. responds to penicillin

Q.9.8   Tumours of vascular origin include

a. glomus tumour
b. pyogenic granuloma
c. Kaposi's sarcoma
d. cellular naevi
e. milia

Q.9.9   Topical antisepsis may be achieved by the use of

a. povidone-iodine
b. triclosan
c. terfenadine
d. clioquinol
e. salicylic acid

Q.9.10   Psoriasis responds to treatment with

a. benzyl benzoate lotion
b. coal tar preparations
c. dithranol paste
d. UVA irradiation
e. systemic cyclosporin

For answers see over

Answers

A.9.6 a. F
b. F
c. T
d. F
e. T

A.9.7 a. F
b. T—This is due to streptococci.
c. F
d. T—Long-term prophylactic antibiotics may be necessary to prevent this happening.
e. T

A.9.8 a. T—A tumour of the arteriolar muscles and nerves.
b. T—An extremely rapid proliferation of new capillaries.
c. T—A malignant angiosarcoma.
d. F—Common moles.
e. F—Small intraepidermal keratin cysts.

A.9.9 a. T—Betadine is one example.
b. T—Sterzac is one example.
c. F—This is an antihistamine.
d. T—Often in combination with steroids, e.g. Betnovate C.
e. F—This is a keratolytic.

A.9.10 a. F—This is the treatment for scabies.
b. T
c. T
d. F—Sensitisation with psoralens is required as well (PUVA).
e. T—But hardly first-line treatment!

Q.9.11 **Discoid lupus erythematosus**

    a. usually develops into systemic lupus erythematosus
    b. may produce scarring alopecia
    c. is improved by sunlight or UVB
    d. may be treated with hydroxychloroquine
    e. frequently affects the kidneys

Q.9.12 **Regarding the case of a young man who suffered from an episode of malaise followed by a rash consisting of "target" lesions on the extremities and ulcers in the mouth:**

    a. This history is suggestive of lichen planus
    b. The malaise is most likely to have been due to a viral infection
    c. Drugs may have caused the problem
    d. The eruption will settle within 24 hours on topical steroid therapy
    e. A recurrence is unlikely

Q.9.13 **The cutaneous features of sarcoidosis include**

    a. granulomata occurring in old scars
    b. the Köbner phenomenon
    c. lupus pernio
    d. erythema multiforme
    e. poor wound healing

Q.9.14 **Lichen planus**

    a. can affect just the oral mucosa
    b. is characterised by Wickham's striae
    c. tends to pick out the extensor aspect of the wrists
    d. can be caused by drugs
    e. responds poorly to topical steroids

Q.9.15 **Distortion of the nails may result from**

    a. peritonitis
    b. lichen planus
    c. epidermolysis bullosa simplex
    d. eczema
    e. cryotherapy near the nail

For answers see over

Answers

A.9.11 a. F—It is usually a separate condition.
      b. T
      c. F—Almost invariably the condition is worse in the summer.
      d. T—This helps the photosensitivity but cannot be continued indefinitely.
      e. F

A.9.12 a. F—This history is characteristic of erythema multiforme.
      b. T—Viral infections are the commonest cause, particularly herpes simplex.
      c. T—An alternative cause.
      d. F—The response to steroids, both topical and systemic, is poor.
      e. F—Recurrent herpes may give recurrent erythema multiforme.

A.9.13 a. T
      b. F
      c. T
      d. F—But erythema nodosum does occur.
      e. F

A.9.14 a. T—It may present to dentists in this way.
      b. T—These are virtually pathognomonic.
      c. F—The flexor aspects of the wrists are affected.
      d. T
      e. T—Systemic steroids may be required for severe attacks.

A.9.15 a. T—Transverse Beau's lines may follow any debilitating illness.
      b. T—Sometimes this causes pterygium.
      c. F—But it does result from more serious forms of epidermolysis bullosa.
      d. T—When it affects the area of the nailfold.
      e. T—This is a trap for the unwary.

Q.9.16 **In a 30-year-old woman complaining of hair loss it could be relevant that she**

a. has had a recent pregnancy
b. is hyperthyroid
c. has recently had pityriasis rosea
d. has received methotrextae for the treatment of psoriasis
e. has had a recent permanent wave

Q.9.17 **Allergic contact dermatitis is a frequent problem in the following occupations:**

a. Hairdresser
b. Builder
c. Coal miner
d. Housewife
e. Florist

Q.9.18 **Psoriasis**

a. shows parakeratosis histologically
b. is rarer in blacks than in Caucasians
c. is commoner in Mongoloid races than in Caucasians
d. is associated with onychomycosis
e. may show pinpoint haemorrhages

Q.9.19 **Tinea pedis**

a. is rare before puberty
b. may be caused by *Trichophyton rubrum*
c. responds well to preparations containing clioquinol
d. can be treated with benzyl benzoate
e. is rarely absent if tinea unguium is present

Q.9.20 **Melanocytes**

a. are absent in albinism
b. cease to function in vitiligo
c. are of neural crest origin
d. are more numerous in deeply pigmented skin
e. are dendritic

For answers see over

Answers

A.9.16 a. T—Telogen effluvium is common.

      b. T—Slight thinning of the hair occurs in about 50% of cases.

      c. F

      d. F—The dose of this cytotoxic agent is too small to cause hair loss.

      e. T—Damage to the keratin may cause traumatic loss.

A.9.17 a. F—Irritant is much more frequent.

      b. T—Usually chromate in cement is responsible.

      c. F—Irritant is much more frequent.

      d. F—Irritant is much more frequent.

      e. T

A.9.18 a. T—Seen histologically as retention of the nuclei in stratum corneum cells.

      b. T

      c. F—It is rarer.

      d. F—It is associated with onycholysis.

      e. T—This appearance is known as the Auspitz sign.

A.9.19 a. T—Eruptions on the feet in children are rarely fungal.

      b. T—This is the commonest organism.

      c. F—Clioquinol is a useful antiseptic active against candida but not dermatophytes.

      d. F—Benzoic acid (contained in Whitfield's ointment) is mildly antifungal.

      e. T—It is the usual source of the original infection of the nails.

A.9.20 a. F—They are present in normal numbers but are tyrosinase deficient.

      b. F—They are absent in the affected areas.

      c. T

      d. F—The numbers are the same but they are functionally more active.

      e. T—The dendrites pass between the keratinocytes.

Paper 10

Q.10.1 The following fungi are recognised causes of tinea pedis:

a. *Trichophyton rubrum*
b. *Agaricus campestris*
c. *Trichophyton verrucosum*
d. *Epidermophyton floccosum*
e. *Microsporum audouinii*

Q.10.2 There is malignant potential in

a. senile lentigines
b. basal cell papillomata
c. Bowen's disease
d. solar keratoses
e. chondrodermatitis helicis

Q.10.3 Pemphigus

a. may present as oral ulcers
b. may show a positive Nikolski sign
c. is fatal if untreated
d. usually responds to prednisolone in a dose of 20–40 mg daily
e. is the commonest primary blistering disorder

Q.10.4 In photobiology

a. UVC is defined as short wave ultraviolet that is screened out by ozone
b. visible light ranges from 400–760 nm
c. no dermatoses are affected adversely by the visible wavelengths of light
d. UVA has no effect on the normal skin
e. the burning rays of natural sunlight are UVB

Q.10.5 Penile lesions are frequent in

a. lichen planus
b. discoid lupus erythematosus
c. scabies
d. Kaposi's sarcoma
e. lichen sclerosus et atrophicus

For answers see over

Answers

A.10.1 a. T—The commonest cause.
           b. F—The common field mushroom.
           c. F—This fungus causes cattle ringworm, which may affect humans and cause a kerion.
           d. T—But not as common as 40 years ago.
           e. F—This fungus causes scalp ringworm in children.

A.10.2 a. F
           b. F—Synonym is seborrhoeic warts.
           c. T—A form of intraepidermal squamous cell carcinoma.
           d. T—A form of intraepidermal squamous cell carcinoma.
           e. F—A totally benign if painful condition.

A.10.3 a. T—Sometimes mouth ulceration occurs a few months before cutaneous lesions appear.
           b. T—Especially in the "foliaceous" form.
           c. T
           d. F—Much higher doses are usually required.
           e. F—It is rare.

A.10.4 a. T
           b. T
           c. F—Porphyria is one example.
           d. F—UVA causes slight tanning (immediate pigment darkening).
           e. T

A.10.5 a. T
           b. F
           c. T—*Sarcoptes scabiei* is a sexy little beast; it also affects the nipples in women.
           d. F
           e. T—This condition is called balanitis xerotica obliterans.

Q.10.6 Both acne vulgaris and rosacea will respond to treatment with

a. minocycline
b. erythromycin
c. metronidazole
d. retinoids
e. cephalosporins

Q.10.7 Dermatophyte infections may be treated topically with

a. amphotericin
b. mupirocin
c. quinoline derivatives (e.g. clioquinol)
d. imidazoles
e. griseofulvin

Q.10.8 Curettage is satisfactory treatment for

a. benign naevi
b. seborrhoeic keratoses
c. basal cell carcinomata
d. keratoacanthomata
e. pyogenic granuloma

Q.10.9 The cutaneous manifestations of systemic lupus erythematosus include

a. nailfold telangiectasia
b. light sensitivity
c. hair loss
d. pinpoint periungual infarcts
e. Raynaud's phenomenon

Q.10.10 Streptococcal infections may give rise to

a. erythema multiforme
b. erythema nodosum
c. erysipeloid
d. anaphylactoid purpura
e. Hand-foot-and-mouth disease

For answers see over

Answers

A.10.6 a. T—All tetracycline derivatives are helpful.
          b. F—Acne only will respond.
          c. F—Rosacea only will respond.
          d. F—There is a minimal response in rosacea.
          e. F—Neither responds well.

A.10.7 a. F—This is only effective against candida infections.
          b. F—This is pseudomonic acid, a topical antibiotic mainly effective against Gram-positive organisms.
          c. F—These are only effective against candida and bacterial infections.
          d. T—Most of the commonly used preparations (e.g. clotrimazole, miconazole, sulconazole) are in this group.
          e. F—This is only effective systemically.

A.10.8 a. F—These lesions are too fibrotic.
          b. T—These are very superficial tumours.
          c. F—Clearance cannot be guaranteed.
          d. T—But be sure of the diagnosis.
          e. T

A.10.9 a. T—This may sometimes be the only cutaneous feature.
          b. T—This accounts for the butterfly eruption.
          c. T
          d. F—These are characteristic of rheumatoid arthritis.
          e. T

A.10.10 a. F
           b. T
           c. F—Erysipeloid is caused by *Erysipelothrix rhusiopathiae*. (Erysipe*las* is a synonym for cellulitis.)
           d. T—Synonym is Henoch–Schönlein purpura.
           e. F—This is caused by a Coxsackie virus, usually A16.

Q.10.11 The clinical features of Behçet's disease include

    a. arthritis
    b. colitis
    c. oral ulcers
    d. keratoderma blenorrhagica
    e. optic neuritis

Q.10.12 Pityriasis rosea

    a. causes patchy hypo- or hyperpigmentation depending on light exposure
    b. affects the palms and soles in particular
    c. characteristically fades leaving a herald spot
    d. is often recurrent
    e. mostly affects younger adults

Q.10.13 A 14-year-old boy develops blisters on his legs after a summer's day spent playing in a field. These lesions might arise from

    a. plant photo-contact dermatitis
    b. discoid lupus erythematosis (DLE)
    c. papular urticaria
    d. epidermolysis bullosa simplex
    e. erythropoietic protoporphyria

Q.10.14 The beard area in the male might be specifically affected in

    a. acne keloid
    b. sycosis barbae
    c. alopecia areata
    d. pseudofolliculitis
    e. *Trichophyton verrucosum* infection

Q.10.15 Excessive hair loss is found

    a. in anorexia nervosa
    b. with minoxidil therapy
    c. during pregnancy
    d. in hypothyroidism
    e. during contraceptive pill therapy

For answers see over

Answers

A.10.11 a. T

   b. F

   c. T—Usually mouth ulcers are the presenting and dominant feature.

   d. F—This is a feature of Reiter's disease.

   e. T—In addition to the commoner uveitis.

A.10.12 a. F—Hypo- or hyperpigmentation are features of pityriasis *versicolor*.

   b. F—It is central in distribution.

   c. F—It *starts* with a herald patch.

   d. F—Rarely if ever do second attacks occur.

   e. T

A.10.13 a. T—Many plants contain psoralens or other photosensitisers.

   b. F—Sunlight is a triggering cause of DLE, but the site and age are wrong.

   c. T—Insect bites are the most likely cause.

   d. F—The lesions would be at sites of trauma on the feet.

   e. F—This condition mainly affects the face and hands, and the symptoms are immediate, requiring a cessation of activities.

A.10.14 a. F—Usually affects the nape of the neck in blacks.

   b. T—Folliculitis of the coarse terminal hairs.

   c. T

   d. T—Repenetration by hairs growing at an acute angle.

   e. T—Cattle ringworm of the terminal hairs.

A.10.15 a. F—An increase in vellus hair is usual.

   b. F—Hypertrichosis may be a problem.

   c. F—A telogen effluvium may occur 3 months *after* childbirth.

   d. T

   e. F

Q.10.16 Allergic contact dermatitis is commonly caused by

    a. chromate
    b. gold wedding rings
    c. compositae
    d. epoxy resins
    e. industrial cutting oils

Q.10.17 Psoriasis could reasonably be treated with topical dithranol in a concentration of

    a. 0.001%
    b. 0.01%
    c. 0.1%
    d. 1.0%
    e. 10%

Q.10.18 Basal cell carcinomata

    a. occur only on light-exposed skin
    b. show the same distribution as squamous cell carcinomata
    c. can be fatal
    d. may be associated with internal malignancy
    e. may arise from an epidermal naevus

Q.10.19 Bleeding may be a prominent feature of

    a. pyogenic granulomata
    b. capillary naevi
    c. cavernous haemangiomata
    d. Campbell de Morgan spots
    e. malignant melanomata

Q.10.20 It is true to state that

    a. candida intertrigo can be treated with amphotericin B topically
    b. pityriasis rosea is a fungal infection caused by *Pityrosporum orbiculare* (*Malassezia furfur*)
    c. griseofulvin is an effective treatment for candidiasis
    d. *Candida albicans* infections are more common in patients with diabetes mellitus
    e. erythrasma can be identified with the aid of Wood's light.

For answers see over

Answers

A.10.16 a. T—Often from handling cement or leather.
  b. F—Wedding ring dermatitis is due to trapped detergent residues.
  c. T—Chrysanthemum is one member of this plant family.
  d. T—Before they harden.
  e. F—These usually produce an irritant reaction.

A.10.17 a. F
  b. F
  c. T
  d. T
  e. F—The maximum concentration is usually about 5% or less, depending on the base.

A.10.18 a. F—But they usually do.
  b. F—There are differences with squamous cell carcinomata, which are more directly linked to light exposure.
  c. T—As a result of infection or erosion of a major vessel.
  d. F
  e. F—At any time during adult life.

A.10.19 a. T—Usually bleeding is the presenting feature.
  b. F—It is surprisingly rare.
  c. T—But only in the early stages.
  d. F
  e. T—It may be an early feature.

A.10.20 a. T—Amphotericin is closely related to nystatin.
  b. F—This fungus causes pityriasis *versicolor*.
  c. F—Only dermatophyte infections respond.
  d. T
  e. T—It fluoresces coral pink.

Batch number: 09635029

Printed by Printforce, the Netherlands